Hydrogen Peroxide Handbook

Proven Secrets to Optimum Health, Quick Healing, Illness Prevention and Natural Beauty

by Jessica Jacobs

Copyright © 2014 by Jessica Jacobs

All rights reserved. No part of this book may be reproduced in any form without permission in writing from the author. Reviewers are able to quote brief passages in reviews.

Disclaimer

This document is geared towards providing exact and reliable information in regards to the topic and issue covered. The publication is sold with the idea that the publisher is not required to render accounting, officially permitted, or otherwise, qualified services. If advice is necessary, legal or professional, a practiced individual in the profession should be ordered.

- From a Declaration of Principles which was accepted and approved equally by a Committee of the American Bar Association and a Committee of Publishers and Associations.

In no way is it legal to reproduce, duplicate, or transmit any part of this document in either electronic means or in printed format. Recording of this publication is strictly prohibited and any storage of this document is not allowed unless with written permission from the publisher. All rights reserved.

The information provided herein is stated to be truthful and consistent, in that any liability, in terms of inattention or otherwise, by any usage or abuse of any policies, processes, or directions contained within is the solitary and utter responsibility of the recipient reader. Under no circumstances will any legal responsibility or blame be held against the publisher for any reparation, damages, or monetary loss due to the information herein, either directly or indirectly.

Respective authors own all copyrights not held by the publisher.

The information herein is offered for informational purposes solely, and is universal as so. The presentation of the information is without contract or any type of guarantee assurance.

The trademarks that are used are without any consent, and the publication of the trademark is without permission or backing by the trademark owner. All trademarks and brands within this book are for clarifying purposes only and are the owned by the owners themselves, not affiliated with this document.

About This Book

This book aims to introduce you to hydrogen peroxide and its home use for various applications. It's informational and to the point, and divided into sections on using hydrogen peroxide for healthcare, beauty, cleaning and gardening to let you get the full range of benefits from this versatile compound. Each section is complete with the needed information, and a chapter on safety tips and techniques is also included.

You will find concluding remarks and a list of additional resources at the end of this book. I will also give you a preview of another book of mine which I am sure will delight you as well.

The following table of contents will show you exactly what is covered in this book.

Table of Contents

Introduction 1
Chapter 1: What Is an Element? 3
   Metals and Non-Metals 4
Chapter 2: What Is a Molecule? 6
Chapter 3: Hydrogen Peroxide 8
   Discovery of Hydrogen Peroxide 8
   Structure and Chemical Properties of Hydrogen Peroxide ... 9
   Preparation of Hydrogen Peroxide 11
   Functions of Hydrogen Peroxide 11
Chapter 4: Differences between Hydrogen Peroxide and Water 13
   Physical properties 14
   Thermodynamic properties 15
   Electrical properties 16
   Radiation properties 16
Chapter 5: Applications of Hydrogen Peroxide 18
   Industrial applications 18
   Agricultural Application 18
   Medical Applications 19
      Disinfection 19
      In Cosmetics 19
      In alternative medicine 19
   Other Applications 20
Chapter 6: Facts about Hydrogen Peroxide 22
Chapter 7: Health Benefits of Hydrogen Peroxide 26

Health Applications of Hydrogen Peroxide 26

Detoxification Using Hydrogen Peroxide Bath Therapy 28

Disease Prevention 29

Chapter 8: Beauty Benefits of Hydrogen Peroxide 32

Hair 32

Ears / Nose / Throat 34

Face/ Skin 36

Mouth and Teeth 37

Personal Hygiene 37

Nails 37

Chapter 9: Home Benefits of Hydrogen Peroxide 38

General Home Uses 38

Kitchen Uses 39

Garden Uses 41

Effects on Plant Health 43

Chapter 10: Cool Experiments with Hydrogen Peroxide 45

Detection of fingerprints using hydrogen peroxide and vinegar 45

Reaction of hydrogen peroxide with blood 46

Hydrogen peroxide hybrid rocket 47

Making an oxygen balloon with hydrogen peroxide 49

Explosive decomposition of hydrogen peroxide 51

Elephant toothpaste 52

The color-changing rose 54

Chapter 11: Precautions and Safe Practices 56

Grades of Hydrogen Peroxide 56

Dilution of Hydrogen Peroxide 57

Storage and Decomposition of Hydrogen Peroxide............ 59

First Aid 61

Firefighting Measures Related to Hydrogen Peroxide........ 62

Conclusion 64

Key Takeaways... 65

How to Put This Information into Action 66

Resources for Further Reading and Viewing 70

Preview of Natural Remedies that Work: How to Heal and Protect Yourself without the Use of Prescription 72

More Books You Might Like.. 83

Your Free Bonus 84

Introduction

First, I would like to express my sincere gratitude to you for taking the time to download this e-book. I assure you that all the insight you will gain from this comprehensive text will serve to increase your overall knowledge and leave you feeling that you've made a very wise purchase.

The main reason I wrote this text was to provide readers with in-depth knowledge of the many applications of the hydrogen peroxide compound. Most of these don't require a lot of expertise about the chemical components of this compound, although I've included that information as well for those who are interested. This *Hydrogen Peroxide Handbook* is dedicated to both ordinary individuals who want to find out a little bit about hydrogen peroxide and people who already have some basic knowledge about it and want to learn more. In addition, it is also dedicated to professionals who use it in their work in the hope that the supplementary knowledge they gain will come in handy for their particular applications. This handbook is written with a sense of gratitude for the discovery of hydrogen peroxide and its many beneficial uses.

With the other readers of this book, you will learn many interesting facts about the only germicidal agent that is composed of only hydrogen and oxygen. A wide range of information about the properties of hydrogen peroxide will show you its importance and its uses in simple yet crucial aspects of everyday life that you probably never knew of or thought about before.

That information is presented in a logical order, starting from hydrogen peroxide's chemical composition and continuing through its health, beauty, and home benefits all the way up to the safety precautions for handling this compound. In addition, possible side effects of hydrogen peroxide use are extensively detailed to give you a clear and objective view of all the issues.

This text covers both domestic and industrial applications of hydrogen peroxide, thereby helping you fully appreciate how important the compound is in modern society. You'll also find out how much hydrogen peroxide has helped in technological development since its isolation in the late nineteenth century.

This *Hydrogen Peroxide Handbook* contains little-known techniques for using hydrogen peroxide to deal with a variety of problems – both minor and significant – that you encounter in your day-to-day activities. Your attentive reading of this text will leave you with a refined understanding of all of the many applications of hydrogen peroxide.

Chapter 1:
What Is an Element?

An element is a pure substance composed of a single type of atoms (atoms are the building blocks of any substance). Each element is differentiated from other elements due to its atomic weight, number of protons and electrons, and many other chemical properties like color, reactivity with other chemicals, etc.

Humans have identified 118 elements, most of which are natural and some of which are manmade. These elements are the basis of everything on earth: from the biggest blue whale to the smallest needle, everything has these elements in it.

Every atom of every element is made from smaller units called electrons, protons, and neutrons. Electrons are negatively charged and have the smallest mass and size. Protons are positively charged and have a considerable mass that is approximately 2,000 times the mass of electrons. Neutrons, as the name implies, are neutral, having neither positive nor negative charge, but they are heavier and larger than both electrons and protons. Even though electrons are the smallest, they play a major role in many chemical phenomena.

For our convenience, elements are grouped in a tabular format called the periodic table. The periodic table has 7 rows and 18 columns. Rows are called periods and columns are called groups.

Every element of the periodic table is represented by a letter or two from the Greek or Latin name of the element. They are also described with a specific atomic mass and atomic number.

The atomic number of an element is the number of protons in the element, and the atomic mass is effectively the sum of the mass of the protons and neutrons together (the electrons are light enough to be discounted).

The periodic table has elements arranged from lightest to heaviest. The lightest element is and the heaviest element is ununoctium.

Not all the elements are solid; they can be solids, liquids or gasses depending upon their temperature and many other factors like pressure, solubility etc. Though the atoms of all elements are similar in shape, they have different chemical and physical properties because of their interactions and reactions with other elements.

Usually, those elements that are solids at standard ambient temperature and pressure (SATP), where temperature is 25 degrees Celsius and absolute pressure is 100 kPa, have high affinity towards other atoms of the same element.

Those elements that are liquid at SATP also have relatively high affinity between atoms of the same element, but not enough to keep them solid. Those elements that are gasses at SATP have very weak affinity between the atoms of the same element.

Metals and Non-Metals

Based on their physical and chemical properties, elements are categorized into metals and nonmetals. In layman's terms, metals are elements which conduct electricity, whereas nonmetals cannot or typically do not conduct electricity. This property of electrical conductivity is due to free electrons present in an atom.

Other properties of metals as opposed to nonmetals are that: Metals are malleable (can be beaten into thin, long sheets), but nonmetals are not. Metals are ductile (can be drawn into long sheets), while nonmetals are not. Metals are sonorous (they produce a sharp sound when hit with another hard object; think of a bell), but nonmetals are not. Metals are lustrous (they shine when light falls on them), but nonmetals are not. Almost all metals are solids at room temperature (mercury is the exception), whereas nonmetals are solids, liquids or gasses at room temperature.

On the basis of these basic properties (and some more technical ones) elements are divided into metals and nonmetals. Metals are placed at the left end of the periodic table whereas nonmetals are at the right.

Some classical examples of metals are sodium, iron, gold, silver, platinum, mercury, radium, uranium and so on. Classical examples of nonmetals are carbon, oxygen, sulfur, chlorine, helium, nitrogen and many more.

But there is an element that is neither a metal nor a nonmetal: hydrogen. Hydrogen is not yet classified as a metal or a nonmetal because it exhibits properties of both metals and nonmetals. For example, hydrogen gives electrons to a metal but is a gas. Hence hydrogen is given a special position in the periodic table. Scientists are debating the issue, though, and in the near future it might be classified as a metal or nonmetal.

Chapter 2:
What Is a Molecule?

Atoms tend not to be stable on their own because of their electron configurations. Therefore, they often give or take or share electrons with other atoms and form molecules.

All atoms "want" 8 electrons in their last orbital, which can be thought of as a circular path where electrons revolve around an atom. Atoms that have close to 8 electrons in this orbital (like 7 or 6) prefer to take electrons from other atoms. This is a typical property of nonmetals. If an atom has very few electrons in its last orbital (like 1, 2 or 3) it prefers to give away those electrons to other atoms. This is a typical property of metals.

Hence, if a nonmetal like chlorine has 7 electrons in its last orbital it prefers to take electrons from an element like sodium, which has only one electron in its last orbital. Then the chlorine and sodium atoms form a molecule and both put together have 8 electrons in their last orbitals (7 from chlorine + 1 from sodium = 8 in sodium chloride).

This type of bond between a metal and a nonmetal where electrons are transferred is called an ionic bond. When a bond is formed between two atoms, a molecule is created. A molecule has one or more types of atoms in it.

There are some nonmetals that have 3, 4 or 5 electrons in their last orbital. In these situations nonmetals do not give or take electrons – they share. For example, carbon has four electrons in its last orbital. Hence, it shares its electrons with other carbon molecules or some other nonmetal to maintain stability. This is called a covalent bond.

When two atoms form a molecule, the properties of the atoms are masked and a new set of chemical properties is displayed by the molecule.

Chapter 3:
Hydrogen Peroxide

Hydrogen peroxide in its pure form is a viscous, clear, and unstable liquid that has very powerful oxidizing characteristics. In chemistry, it is a simple compound based on two oxygen atoms bonded together to form a single entity. A compound that consists of two oxygen atoms joined by a single bond is known as a peroxide, and with the addition of a single atom of hydrogen to each of the oxygen atoms, the hydrogen peroxide molecule comes into being.

Discovery of Hydrogen Peroxide

The first production of hydrogen peroxide took place in the early years of the 19th century, in 1818 to be precise, in the laboratory of the eminent French scientist Louis Jacques Thénard. He initially used a reaction of barium peroxide and nitric acid. Later he substituted hydrochloric acid for the nitric acid to come up with a superior version of the procedure, which also involved using sulfuric acid to precipitate the byproduct of the reaction, barium sulfate.

Early attempts to separate hydrogen peroxide from the water that was present in this synthesis were futile, which led to the belief that hydrogen peroxide in its pure form was very unstable. It was later learned that this instability was actually due to the presence of trace contamination that catalyzed the breakdown of the hydrogen peroxide molecules.

Towards the end of the 19th century, in 1984, the distinguished German scientist Richard Wolffenstein made a revolutionary discovery that allowed him to obtain hydrogen peroxide of an impeccable purity level – i.e., 100% pure –

through a vacuum distillation method. A few years later, Petre Melikishvili, a reputable Georgian scientist working in Odessa, Ukraine, together with a student known only as L. Pizarjevski, eliminated numerous proposed formulas for hydrogen peroxide and proved the correct one to be H-O-O-H. Purification and a correct understanding of the structure of hydrogen peroxide led to many ground-breaking scientific innovations related to this versatile compound.

Structure and Chemical Properties of Hydrogen Peroxide

Structure

Hydrogen peroxide is a polar molecule that has a twisted C2 symmetry. The molecule has an atropisomer characteristic, meaning that there is a hindrance of rotation about the single oxygen-oxygen bond due to energy differences resulting from the mutual repulsion between the lone electron pairs of the oxygen atoms.

There is a very distinct structural difference between the crystalline and gaseous forms of hydrogen peroxide. This is because the effect of hydrogen bonding is insignificant in the gaseous state due to the increased distance between molecules. Hydrogen peroxide crystals have a tetragonal shape.

There is an assortment of structural correspondents of hydrogen peroxide, with hydrogen disulfide being the most similar. It has a theoretical boiling point second only to hydrogen peroxide itself, and a fairly high melting point as well. All structurally equivalent compounds display marked thermodynamic instability, especially after exposure to heat, with hydroxylamine and hydrazine most likely to explode. As in hydrogen peroxide, repulsion between lone electron pairs in its analogues dictates a twisted molecular structure.

Properties

- Hydrogen peroxide is a very clear, inorganic, acidic liquid that has no color in its pure form.

- The boiling point of hydrogen peroxide is estimated to be at about 150.2 degrees Celsius, but in the practical sense, it would normally undergo a very explosive and volatile thermal decomposition if exposed to such high temperatures. However, there are a variety of techniques that are used to safely distill it under reduced pressure.

- The properties of aqueous hydrogen peroxide tend to differ from those of the pure form as a result of the changes it undergoes after bonding with water. For instance, its freezing point when combined with water is about -51 degrees Celsius. The boiling point of the combination also ends up being between those of the two components. It is approximately 114 degrees Celsius, which is 14 degrees more than that of pure water and 36.2 degrees less than that of pure hydrogen peroxide.

- Hydrogen peroxide is not highly flammable, but it generates a large amount of oxygen and heat during the decomposition process, which can facilitate combustion.

- Under regular conditions, hydrogen peroxide is extremely stable with evident losses of less than one percent annually under optimum conditions.

- It is among the most powerful oxidizing agents – even more powerful than potassium permanganate, chlorine, and chlorine dioxide – when used in an acidic solution.

- Hydrogen peroxide can also be used in a basic solution as a reducing agent, emitting oxygen as a byproduct.

- It is potentially toxic, and ingestion, inhalation, or contact with the skin or the eyes may lead to severe burns and injury or even death.

- Combustion of hydrogen peroxide may lead to the production of irritating and toxic gases.

Preparation of Hydrogen Peroxide

Initially, hydrogen peroxide was industrially manufactured by the hydrolysis of ammonium persulfate, which was derived from the electrolysis of a solution of ammonium bisulfate and sulfuric acid. Presently, it is almost entirely prepared by the anthraquinone process, which was finalized in 1939 and patented three years later. This involves the reduction of 2-ethylanthraquinone or its 2-amyl derivative followed by autoxidation with environmental oxygen which releases hydrogen peroxide.

Functions of Hydrogen Peroxide

Hydrogen peroxide is used by numerous species to carry out various biological functions; for example, the bombardier beetle uses it along with hydroquinone to ward off predators.

More importantly for our purposes, research has shown that it plays a very important role in the immunity of our bodies. Scientists found significantly increased levels of hydrogen peroxide in the injured tissues of zebra fish, and hypothesized that this signals white blood cells to come together at the site of an injury to initiate the healing process. The researchers proved their hypothesis by showing that when genes responsible for production of hydrogen peroxide were incapacitated, white blood cells did not converge in the region of injury. (The experiment was carried out on fish because of their genetic similarity to humans.)

The same study also indicated that asthma sufferers have elevated levels of hydrogen peroxide in their respiratory systems, which persuasively explains why these individuals also have increased levels of white blood cells in their lungs.

Hydrogen peroxide also plays a crucial part as a signaling molecule for the control of a wide range of biological processes in the human body. And according to the free radical theory of the aging process, the byproducts of cellular metabolism can react with ambient water, leading to formation of hydrogen peroxide. These radicals in turn readily react with components of somatic cells, especially the mitochondria, leading to the destruction of vital cellular constituents.

Chapter 4:
Differences between Hydrogen Peroxide and Water

Though both water and hydrogen peroxide have hydrogen and oxygen in their molecular structure, they have a different ratio of hydrogen to oxygen, i.e., hydrogen peroxide has a ratio of 1:1 whereas water has 1:2 oxygen to hydrogen). They also differ in their molecular structure in terms of their bond angles, bond lengths and bond energies. Hence, they show different properties both physically and chemically.

- Water and hydrogen peroxide are transparent.

- Hydrogen peroxide is more viscous than water.

- Hydrogen peroxide is much denser than water.

- Hydrogen peroxide decomposes while water does not.

- Hydrogen peroxide has a higher boiling point than water.

- Hydrogen peroxide acts as a catalyst in many chemical, biochemical and biological reactions whereas water is a less common catalyst (all biochemical and biological reactions require water, but it is not a catalyst).

- Hydrogen peroxide has a pungent smell but water is odorless.

- Hydrogen peroxide must be stored in dark-colored containers while water can be stored in any container (because hydrogen peroxide is photosensitive but water is not).

- The solubility of water is greater than that of hydrogen peroxide.

Physical properties

- Hydrogen peroxide is soluble in water in all concentrations.

- The specific gravity or density of a hydrogen peroxide mixture increases with an increase in the concentration of hydrogen peroxide in water.

- The vapors of hydrogen peroxide at standard temperature and pressure obey the ideal gas law.

- The thermal expansion coefficient of hydrogen peroxide is greater than that of water.

- Hydrogen peroxide solutions of < 45 wt% expand during freezing, while a solution with concentration > 65% contracts.

- Viscosity of hydrogen peroxide increases with decrease in temperature and is reduced by an increase in temperature.

- Surface tension of hydrogen peroxide increases with decrease in temperature and increase in concentration. It decreases with an increase in the temperature and decrease in concentration.

- The coefficient of diffusion for hydrogen peroxide vapors is 0.189 cm²/sec

- (in air, 60 °C, 1 atm).

- Like water, hydrogen peroxide freezes and melts at 0 degrees Celsius and boils at 100 degrees Celsius.

- Heat of fusion of hydrogen peroxide is 87.84 Cal/gm = 2,987 Cal/mole = 367.64 kJ/kg (at melting point).

- The partial and total vapor pressures of hydrogen peroxide increase with temperature.

- The heat of vaporization of hydrogen peroxide is around 350 Cal/gm at the concentration of 100% wt.

- The heat capacity of hydrogen peroxide liquid is 1 Cal/gm Celsius at 0% concentration and 0.6 Cal/gm Celsius at 100% concentration.

Thermodynamic properties

- The bond angles of hydrogen peroxide are 95 degrees and 120 degrees.

- Bond length of the O-H bond is 0.097 nm and bond length of O-O is 0.149 nm.

- The dipole moment of hydrogen peroxide is 2.2 debyes.

- The heat capacity value for liquid anhydrous hydrogen peroxide over the temperature range of 0-27 °C is 0.628 cal/gm°C.

- The effect of dilution of hydrogen peroxide with water is mildly exothermic (negative ΔH_1) for all concentrations at a temperature of > 21 °C. Some dilution processes below this temperature are endothermic.

- The standard free energy change (Δ Fo) is -27.92 kcal/mole at 25 °C.

- Rapid decomposition of the concentrated hydrogen peroxide solution may not be complete, with concentrations up to 10% remaining.

Electrical properties

- The conductivity of hydrogen peroxide depends on the purity of the sample.

- Like water, hydrogen peroxide is a very weak electrolyte. It has an electrical conductivity that is very similar to that of water.

- The dielectric constant of water is greater than that of hydrogen peroxide at all temperatures.

- A maximum value occurs at about 55 wt. % concentration of hydrogen peroxide at 0 °C, and this value is just 8% to 9% greater than that of water.

- The maximum is more pronounced and shifts to a higher value of hydrogen peroxide concentration as the temperature decreases.

- Like water, hydrogen peroxide is a diamagnetic substance.

Radiation properties

- The refractive index for hydrogen peroxide is greater than the refractive index of water, and the curve relating to the composition of hydrogen peroxide is slightly concave upward.

- Like water, hydrogen peroxide and its solutions are not optically active and no rotation of the plane of polarization is found when light passes through them.

- If a substance containing hydrogen peroxide is illuminated with monochromatic light (light containing a single wavelength or single color), the radiation scattered by the substance is composed not only of the exciting wavelength, but also one or more other wavelengths independent of the exciting wavelength.

- For practical purposes, all solutions of hydrogen peroxide are transparent for radiation to which the eye is sensitive (that is, between 400 and 800 nanometers).

- In bulk solutions, however, hydrogen peroxide will appear slightly pale blue with a tinge of green.

- The yellow to green tint is attributed to light scattering due to entrapped bubbles, whereas the blue colored note is similar to that seen in the water.

Chapter 5:
Applications of Hydrogen Peroxide

Industrial applications

- Approximately three-fifths of the hydrogen peroxide produced in the world is applied to the bleaching of pulp and paper.

- The second most significant industrial application of hydrogen peroxide is in the production of the mild bleaches present in laundry detergents.

- It is also used in polymerization, for bleaching flour, and as an acne treatment method.

- Hydrogen peroxide is used in the process of water treatment to get rid of organic contaminants and impurities by the processes of advanced oxidation. This can also help in the reduction of odor.

Agricultural Application

- Some horticultural specialists support the use of a weak solution of hydrogen peroxide mixed with water. Its spontaneous decomposition leads to the release of oxygen that boosts the development of plant roots. It also assists in the treatment of root rot resulting from insufficient oxygen in the roots.

Medical Applications

Disinfection

- Hydrogen peroxide is regarded as an environmentally friendly alternative to chlorine-based bleaches. It can be effectively applied on various surfaces for thorough disinfection. It is a recognized, FDA-approved antimicrobial agent that is generally recognized as safe.

- It has been used as a wound disinfectant from the beginning of its industrial production due to its low cost and ready availability in comparison to other antiseptics. In fact, a single application at a very low concentration is thought to induce the process of healing.

In Cosmetics

- In dilutions ranging from 8% to 3% it can be used in the bleaching of human hair when mixed with ammonium hydroxide.

- It is also commonly applied as a tool for teeth whitening in dentistry, and can even be combined with salt and baking soda to come up with simple homemade toothpaste.

- Hydrogen peroxide is sometimes used in the treatment of acne.

In alternative medicine

- More and more alternative medicine practitioners have come out in favor of the use of hydrogen peroxide in the treatment of a very wide variety of conditions which include influenza, emphysema, and even HIV/AIDS. It has also reportedly been used in the treatment of certain cancers. In this case hydrogen peroxide is either consumed orally or administered by injection. This is based upon two main guiding principles: first, that the body tends produces hydrogen peroxide to naturally fight infections; second, that the pathogens that affect the human body cannot exist in environments that are very rich in oxygen. It is therefore believed that either the ingestion or the injection of hydrogen peroxide kills infections by increasing the levels of oxygen in the body and simultaneously imitating the body's natural immune response. However, those who disagree point out that the body itself releases hydrogen peroxide in very limited, harmless amounts, and it is also enclosed in compartments referred to as phagosomes, as it is likely to harm the cells as well as invading pathogens. Free hydrogen peroxide present in the human body can lead to tissue damage.

Other Applications

There are an immense number of uses of hydrogen peroxide apart from those detailed above. Some of them include:

- As a propellant in the propulsion system of a rocket.

- In the creation of explosives that are based on the organic peroxides, for instance acetone peroxide, for IED (Improvised Explosive Device) applications.

- In domestic settings, hydrogen peroxide can be used as both a disinfectant and a cleaning agent

- It is reacted with other compounds in order generate the light in the much-adored glow sticks.

Scientific tests have confirmed that the conventional hydrogen peroxide used for domestic purposes can be safely used to provide a supply of oxygen to aquarium fish. This is because it releases oxygen in the decomposition process upon exposure to catalysts such as manganese dioxide.

Chapter 6:
Facts about Hydrogen Peroxide

- Hydrogen peroxide is found in all living organisms.

- In humans, hydrogen peroxide is produced by erythrocytes or white blood cells (WBC) to fight against pathogens like bacteria, algae and viruses.

- Plants also produce hydrogen peroxide.

- Fruits and vegetables contain hydrogen peroxide, and this is one of the reasons why eating leafy vegetables and fruits is healthy.

- Amazingly, hydrogen peroxide is found in breast milk. This travels into the baby's system and provides it with an immunity boost to fight against pathogens.

- Hydrogen peroxide makes plants grow faster than normal water (if given in proper amounts).

- Rainwater also contains traces of hydrogen peroxide. It is formed when water molecules in the rain take extra oxygen from the ozone layer. This is the reason why trees are taller in regions with high rainfall and a thick ozone layer.

- Hydrogen peroxide is used as a supply of oxygen to burn fuel in rockets.

- Hydrogen peroxide eliminates the harmful effects of chlorine in chlorine-treated water.

- The concentrated form of hydrogen peroxide is used as an explosive.

- Hydrogen peroxide can be a hazardous substance; it is listed on the special health hazard substance list.

- Hydrogen peroxide can be very dangerous to one's health if inhaled. It primarily causes choking and irritation in the throat and nose. If inhaled in higher amounts for a long period of time it can cause pulmonary edema, a very serious medical emergency.

- Hydrogen peroxide is a mutagen (known to cause cancer) and must be handled with care.

- Exposure to hydrogen peroxide causes nausea, dizziness, vomiting and headache.

- Though hydrogen peroxide is used in explosives, it does not burn; rather it is a strong oxidizing agent that enhances the combustion of other substances.

- If hydrogen peroxide is in contact with air, it may cause severe eye damage and lead to blindness.

- Hydrogen peroxide has the potential to cause reproductive harm.

- Hydrogen peroxide is used to sanitize meat prior to cooking.

- The hydrogen peroxide sold in neighborhood drugstores and supermarkets is only 3.5 % concentration, and is assumed to be pharmaceutical grade.

- Usually, pharmaceutical grade hydrogen peroxide contains assorted stabilizers that should not be ingested. These stabilizers include acetanilide, phenol, sodium stagnate and tetrasodium phosphate.

- A concentration of 6% hydrogen peroxide is beautician grade. This is usually used in saloons to dye hair and treat pimples. This is not for internal use.

- A concentration of 30% hydrogen peroxide is reagent grade. This is only used in scientific experiments and also contains stabilizers; hence it should not be ingested.

- A concentration of 32% hydrogen peroxide is electronic grade and can be used for cleaning electronic items (but not for internal use).

- A concentration of 35% hydrogen peroxide is food grade and is used for producing cheese, cleansing eggs and also in the purification and decontamination of milk products.

- Food grade hydrogen peroxide is used for spraying on foil linings to maintain aseptic conditions and is the only type of hydrogen peroxide that should be used for internal purposes.

- Even food grade hydrogen peroxide can be extremely harmful since it is a strong oxidizer. If it is not diluted, it is extremely dangerous or fatal.

- Any concentration of hydrogen peroxide above 10 % (even food grade) is very dangerous and can lead to neurological disorders and injure the upper gastrointestinal track.

- Hydrogen is a well-known and efficient antiseptic for small wounds. This ability of hydrogen peroxide is due to its ability to decompose; as it decomposes it forms nascent oxygen, which in turn reacts with the proteins of pathogens and degrades them, leading to the death of pathogens.

- To get a classic sun-bleached look for your hair, simply spray hydrogen peroxide over moist hair and let it soak for a minimum of 10 to 15 minutes before rinsing out.

- Put fingertips or toes in 3 % solution of hydrogen peroxide to naturally whiten fingernails and toenails.

- Hydrogen is peroxide is well known to remove corns. Make a 50- 50 solution of hydrogen peroxide in water and soak the affected feet. For best results do this twice or thrice a day. If it causes irritation, discontinue.

Chapter 7:
Health Benefits of Hydrogen Peroxide

Food grade hydrogen peroxide is a specially purified and refined form of hydrogen peroxide that is completely safe for consumption. In fact, the hydrogen peroxide easily available in drug stores and meant for application on external wounds and infections is not in any way dangerous for internal consumption. Hydrogen peroxide is an exceptionally powerful antimicrobial, especially when it comes to bacteria, and it has the ability to oxidize a wide range of unwanted substances. There are numerous uncontested health benefits associated with hydrogen peroxide, while there are others whose status is somewhat controversial.

Health Applications of Hydrogen Peroxide

Remedies

Hydrogen peroxide can be used in singlet oxygen therapy because it can release a single oxygen atom upon contact with other elements in an oxidation reaction. After the release of the oxygen atom, the remainder of the hydrogen peroxide molecule disintegrates and breaks down to form water. The single oxygen atom that is released into the body is very reactive and can oxidize or reduce the molecular structure of any undesirable organisms or compounds present in the body – for instance, parasites, fungi, bacteria, and foreign proteins. It can also oxidize or reduce any tissue that has been affected by disease or infection. This atomic oxygen, O_1, has a very high energy and an enhanced capacity for healing as compared to the atmospheric oxygen, O_2, which humans normally breathe.

First Aid and External Contamination

Hydrogen peroxide is probably most popular for its strong capabilities in disinfecting minor cuts and treating minor infections. Standard food grade concentrations are safe for such external application, despite the fact that they are often sold in rather higher concentrations than drug store hydrogen peroxide. For instance, conventional drug store hydrogen peroxide is diluted to about 3.5 percent, whereas food grade offerings have a range of between 8 to 35 percent. Food grade hydrogen peroxide is thus likely to cause a slight tingling or burning sensation upon application to an open wound. However, this does not mean that it will cause severe damage, or indeed any damage whatsoever, to healthy, functioning tissue. According to Biochemical, Physiological, and Molecular Aspects of Human Nutrition by Dr. Martha H. Stipanuk, hydrogen peroxide has the ability to damage and destroy virtually all harmful pathogens upon contact.

Oral Health and Nourishment

Food grade hydrogen peroxide has a very significant effect on your teeth. It is not harmful and does not have to be diluted to a lower concentration; there is absolutely no need to be afraid of using it. It may lead to a rather intense tingling or burning sensation, but also to a potent effect on harmful oral bacteria! In any case, a hydrogen peroxide concentration of 3.5% is all that is really required to put down your oral pathogens. This means you can save money by diluting a sufficient amount of the food grade hydrogen peroxide for daily oral use. A range of proven health benefits are associated with oral use of hydrogen peroxide, including teeth whitening, reduced risk of gum disease, fewer canker sores and cavities, and most obviously, fresher breath.

Detoxification Using Hydrogen Peroxide Bath Therapy

The human body system has the ability to get rid of toxins with the help of four critical organs: the lungs, the kidneys, the skin, and the colon (aided by the liver). A bath of hydrogen peroxide can assist in the cleansing and purification of the skin. This hydrogen peroxide bath helps destroy organisms and toxins, and even reduces the residues that are left after the use of soap.

One of the best things about hydrogen peroxide is that it performs its detoxification function in an environmentally friendly manner: the only byproducts released are oxygen and water. All you need for a hydrogen peroxide bath is a bathtub and two quarts of hydrogen peroxide.

Directions for hydrogen peroxide bath therapy

1. Pour a single quart of hydrogen peroxide into a hot bath. Make sure that you mix it thoroughly to avoid any sort of skin irritation.

2. You should be very careful not to get any water in your eyes, as it might lead to irritation.

3. Fully immerse yourself in the water and then wait for about five minutes.

4. If there is absolutely no noticeable reaction on your skin, you need to add the second quart and stir thoroughly again. Relax and soak for about twenty to twenty-five minutes.

5. You will definitely be amazed by the residue that is left behind after a thorough skin detoxification bath!

6. The efficacy of the bath will be boosted by brushing dry skin all over your body.

Brushing the dry skin gets rid of the layer of dead skin that can be a hindrance to absorption of both nutrients and energy from the bath. The brushing of dry skin also stimulates the lymph fluids and the blood to rise to the skin surface, which the skin to accommodate the healing effects of the hydrogen peroxide bath. For detoxification therapy, take this bath for a minimum of seven successive days, or as recommended by a medical practitioner. However, weekly or even monthly treatments can have a very beneficial effect on your skin nutrition.

Disease Prevention

The antibacterial qualities of hydrogen peroxide make it very suitable for many uses in the improvement of the heath of the human body. Hydrogen peroxide has the ability to fight bacteria, yeast, viruses, and parasites. In fact, quite a number of healthcare professionals have used these advantageous properties of hydrogen peroxide to aid internal parts of the body, for instance the immune system. Medical practitioners have tangible evidence that hydrogen peroxide therapy treatments can have significant positive effects on medical conditions such as human papilloma virus, asthma, degenerative spinal disc disease, leukemia, multiple sclerosis, and arthritis.

The main reason why hydrogen peroxide is applied in the prevention of diseases is the knowledge that infected cells and harmful microorganisms cannot survive in environments that are very rich in oxygen. Since hydrogen peroxide emits oxygen upon its disintegration, once consumed, it is a very efficient supply of oxygen for the internal body systems. This enables the strengthening of the immune system, thereby helping in prevention of diseases and infections.

To treat certain specific infections and prevent them from accelerating, hydrogen peroxide can be consumed in a variety of ways as part of medical hydrogen peroxide therapy. Medical practitioners may suggest its administration either orally or through intravenous injections. Oral administration is simply done by diluting a certain proportion of hydrogen peroxide with water and drinking it.

To prevent diseases at home, you can ensure that all your surfaces are thoroughly cleaned using diluted hydrogen peroxide to get rid of any contamination that might lead to infections. Food-grade hydrogen peroxide can be used to thoroughly clean grocery purchases such as vegetables and fruits. Contaminated vegetables and fruits can lead to chronic stomach upsets if they are not thoroughly disinfected before consumption.

Hydrogen peroxide is also useful in simple health practices – for instance, in the care of your ears to prevent infections, you can use a drop of diluted hydrogen peroxide as a means of softening earwax so you can get rid of any painful or irritating lumps.

Hydrogen peroxide not only offers health benefits to the human body but also presents very real advantages in plant health. If your plants consistently suffer from root rot, hydrogen peroxide is a great remedy. Just apply a solution of thirty parts water to one part hydrogen peroxide at the base of your plants to effectively end the problem. This also encourages root nourishment and development of strong and healthy root systems. Keep applying hydrogen peroxide in this manner to avoid future encounters with root rot.

Chapter 8:
Beauty Benefits of Hydrogen Peroxide

Due to its disinfecting, purifying, and bleaching qualities, hydrogen peroxide is widely used in the formulation and manufacture of cosmetic products, most prevalently in hair care products such as bleaches, dyes, styling solutions, creams and conditioners. It can also be found in teeth bleaching products, toothpaste, and mouthwash. It is also a primary component in solutions used to clean contact lenses, acne treatments, and topical solutions.

Hair

Hydrogen peroxide is an easy and affordable way to lighten your hair or bring out its natural highlights.

You can bleach your hair with products and materials commonly found around the home. You will need 3% hydrogen peroxide solution, a spray bottle, a towel, cotton balls and hair clips. Then, follow these easy steps:

1. Prepare your hair. First, wash it well with shampoo to cleanse it of dirt, oil and residue from other hair products. Doing this allows the hydrogen peroxide to do its job better by eliminating chemical residues that can interfere with its bleaching action. After washing, use an all-natural conditioner to protect your hair from damage such as drying out or breaking during the bleaching process. Pat your hair dry with a towel and allow it to air dry; do not use a blow-dryer. Comb your hair gently. You may begin the bleaching process with damp hair, as hydrogen peroxide work better with hair that is partially wet.

2. Test. First, do a strand test on a small portion from the underside of your hair. Using a cotton ball, gently apply the hydrogen peroxide and allow it to sit for thirty minutes. Rinse the section with cold water and assess for yourself how much peroxide to use. Remember that peroxide has different effects for different hair types.

3. Section. Once you've decided how much to use, begin to section your hair into parts with hair clips or bands, focusing on the areas you want to bleach or highlight. Parting your hair into smaller sections helps achieve a more even color by ensuring that each strand is treated.

4. Bleach. Apply the peroxide to each section using cotton balls in gentle, even strokes from the roots to the tip. You may also want to begin from the bottom and work up to achieve a brighter blond at the tips that gradually fades to dark going toward the roots or as far up your locks as you wish. Repeat this for all the other sections. If you want to bleach all your hair, let down a section at a time and use the spray bottle to spray peroxide on it. Run a comb through the section several times. Repeat with all the other sections. Allow fifteen to thirty minutes for the peroxide to sit on your hair. Assess for yourself how the peroxide works for you in relation to the effect you want to achieve. Remember that the more peroxide you use and the longer you allow it to sit on your hair, the lighter it will be.

5. Wash and style. Rinse off the peroxide thoroughly with cold water. Use a deep moisturizing conditioner, making sure to massage well into your scalp and the roots to repair damage and soothe any irritation and dryness. Rinse well and allow your hair to air dry. Once your hair is dry, style away!

The first time you bleach your hair at home you may not get the exact lightness you wish to achieve. You may need to repeat the process several times until you get exactly what you want.

Treat your bleached hair with extra care. Remember, using peroxide causes dryness and damage. Avoid washing your hair daily, and when you do, allow it to air dry instead of blow-drying. Pat your hair dry instead of wringing or rubbing to keep breakage to a minimum. Avoid hair irons and frequent blow-drying, as this can also contribute to hair damage.

Ears / Nose / Throat

The ears, nose, and throat are all connected. Using hydrogen peroxide solutions on one of them also helps alleviate discomfort and fight infections in the two others.

Ears
Hydrogen peroxide may be used to remove excess ear wax. You will need 3% hydrogen peroxide solution, cotton balls and cotton swabs, a medicine dropper, a towel, and olive oil. Then, follow these easy steps:

1. Warm the olive oil and hydrogen peroxide separately in a warm water bath. Use two to three drops of warm oil in the ear you wish to treat, making sure your head is tilted, with the ear being treated facing up. Take care not to push the dropper too far into the ear canal. Allow a few minutes for the oil to sit in your ear.

2. Next, apply two to three drops of warm hydrogen peroxide in the same ear and let sit for ten to fifteen minutes. You may feel a ticklish sensation and hear bubbles inside your ear. Once the bubbling sensation

has stopped, flip your head over to drain the ear. Use the towel to catch drips and softened ear wax.

3. Do the same for the other ear. You may also use cotton buds or cotton swabs dipped in hydrogen peroxide to clean your outer ear of dirt and oil, taking care not to push the buds deep into your ear canal. Remember to make sure you do not have an existing ear infection or hearing impairment when doing this procedure.

Nose

People with blocked sinuses or stuffy noses due to allergies can do nasal irrigation with a water, salt, and hydrogen peroxide solution to relieve their symptoms. You will need 7 oz. water, 1 oz. 3% hydrogen peroxide, 1 tsp. table salt, a Waterpik® oral irrigator, and a Grossan Hydro Pulse® Sinus System nasal irrigator tip (available at retail stores). Follow these procedures:

1. Mix the water, hydrogen peroxide, and salt and warm the solution by placing it in a warm water bath for a few minutes. Place solution in the Waterpik® with the nasal irrigator tip, making sure the pressure does not push the solution out more than an inch beyond the nasal tip.

2. Place the irrigator tip into one nostril, but not too deep into the nose. Stand over a sink or basin and gently run half of the solution into your nostril while blowing out gently through your mouth. Doing this prevents you from swallowing the solution and allows it to drain out of your other nostril.

3. Repeat the same for the other nostril. You may feel a ticklish and bubbling sensation as you do this. Repeat as necessary in one session, but remember not to do more than two to three irrigation sessions in a day as this may cause drying inside your nose.

Throat

Gargling with hydrogen peroxide can help kill bacteria and relieve sore throat. You will need 3% hydrogen peroxide and warm water. Prepare your gargle solution as follows:

1. Dilute one capful of hydrogen peroxide in one cup of warm water.

2. Gargle with this solution and swish it around your mouth to help kill bacteria in the mouth and on the teeth. Spit out the solution. Take special care not to swallow.

Face/ Skin

Hydrogen peroxide may be used as a detoxifying bath and as a treatment for acne. For a rejuvenating bath, place about two quarts of 3% hydrogen peroxide in your tub of warm water and soak in it for thirty minutes. To treat acne, soak a cotton ball in hydrogen peroxide and gently apply it to the acne breakouts on your face, neck, or back. Let the peroxide stay on your skin for a few minutes or until bubbling stops, then rinse the area thoroughly with water. Use an oil-free facial moisturizer or body lotion to relieve skin dryness. Be careful not to apply hydrogen peroxide too near your eyes, eyelashes, and eyebrows.

Mouth and Teeth

Hydrogen peroxide makes an inexpensive yet effective mouthwash. Use a solution of 3% peroxide and water as your regular mouthwash to help whiten teeth, maintain healthy gums, and alleviate toothache. You can also make your own whitening toothpaste. Add enough peroxide to baking soda to form a paste and use it instead of your regular toothpaste.

Personal Hygiene

Not many people know that hydrogen peroxide can also be used for intimate feminine care as a douche or even as a colonic or enema. For douching, use two cups of 3% hydrogen peroxide in warm water once or twice a week to relieve and prevent yeast infections. For a colonic, use eight ounces of 3% hydrogen peroxide with five gallons of warm water. For an enema, use a solution of one tablespoon 3% peroxide and one quart warm water.

Nails

Hydrogen peroxide is also known to treat nail fungus. Use two ounces of food grade 35% hydrogen peroxide and mix with warm water to use as a finger soak for thirty minutes. You can also use a fifty-fifty hydrogen peroxide and water solution as a spray to cure foot fungus, which can lead to toenail fungus. Repeat three to four times a week or until the infection has cleared. To whiten yellowish nails, you can bleach them using a solution of one tablespoon of 3% hydrogen peroxide and two and a half tablespoons of baking soda. Use cotton swabs to apply the paste to your nails and let sit for three minutes before rinsing with warm water. Do this every six to eight weeks.

Chapter 9:
Home Benefits of Hydrogen Peroxide

Clean surroundings are an important factor in healthy living. A clean home is essential to maintaining our physical and emotional well-being by ensuring we have a safe haven to rest and be comfortable in. A healthy home prevents the spread of infections and diseases and allows us a space to get away from the stress, pollution, and unhealthy conditions of the outside world.

General Home Uses

Well known for its disinfecting, purifying, and bleaching properties, hydrogen peroxide is also an inexpensive, non-toxic, and environmentally friendly solution to cleaning our homes and many of the gadgets we use in them. Unless otherwise specified, all you will need is 3% hydrogen peroxide and water. Scrub and clean away with these easy-to-do methods:

- General Home Disinfectant – Use 3% hydrogen peroxide with water to mop or spray on your floors or wipe down your walls and other home surfaces. Diluted in water, peroxide is completely safe to use, but if you have sensitive skin, you may want to use gloves when handling your solution.

- Laundry – Hydrogen peroxide can also be used when doing your laundry as a safe and effective alternative to bleach. Add a cup of hydrogen peroxide to your load to help brighten white laundry and remove stains and sweat marks. For more effective stain removal, apply some directly on the stain and let it bubble until the stain clears. Repeat as needed. Remember to use it as you would any bleach, keeping coloreds and sensitive materials separated and away from contact.

- Cleaning Applications – Hydrogen peroxide may be used as an all-around cleaning solution for various home appliances, furniture and children's toys, and even for disinfecting your toothbrushes. Make your own all-purpose cleaner with 3% peroxide diluted with water. Put the solution in a spray bottle and you've got yourself a clean-it-all. Spray the solution on whatever it is you're cleaning and wipe down to dry. To disinfect your toothbrushes, bath scrubs, and sponges, soak for a few minutes in a 50-50 peroxide and water solution to clean them of germs and bacteria.

Kitchen Uses

The kitchen is usually the home's most utilized space, and there is no other area where hydrogen peroxide is so useful and versatile as in the kitchen. As the place where we prepare and partake of our food, a consistently clean kitchen is a necessity for good health and overall wellness.

- Food Preparation – You can use hydrogen peroxide when preparing your meals as a safe yet effective fruit and vegetable wash. Keep a spray bottle of 50-50 peroxide and water solution on hand and use it as spray on your kitchen produce. Allow the mix to bubble and do its work for a few minutes, then rinse. This effectively washes away dirt and grime, and also helps remove chemical pesticides and give your produce a longer shelf life.

- Food Storage – Hydrogen peroxide also effectively cleans food storage containers of mildew, fungus, grime, and oils. It is especially effective on plastic storage containers that tend to stain or turn yellow with use over a period of time. Soak your plastic containers in the usual hydrogen peroxide and water solution to disinfect and remove stubborn stains and discoloration. Keeping your food storage containers clean helps ensure your food doesn't get contaminated or spoil so easily.

- Kitchen Cleaning – Use a solution of equal parts of hydrogen peroxide and water as your over-all kitchen cleaner. You can use this to clean your kitchen tiles, counters, under-the-sink area, and garbage bins. To get rid of fungus or mildew, apply hydrogen peroxide directly on the affected area, especially on kitchen tiles, kitchen grout, under the sink, in your pantry, or kitchen cabinets. Let sit for a few minutes and wipe down with water. A word of caution, though: the peroxide might affect the color of some wooden or painted cabinets, so try applying it on an inconspicuous part before using.

Hydrogen peroxide is also very effective for cleaning and disinfecting cutting boards, especially those used for meat and poultry. After washing your board, pour hydrogen peroxide directly on its surface. Treating your board on a regular basis eliminates harmful bacteria like Salmonella and E. coli which often breed on cutting boards and utensils used with infected fish and poultry. Unclean cutting boards are often the cause of food poisoning.

Cleaning your kitchen appliances regularly helps keep them looking new, plus of course eliminates harmful germs that may affect the quality and safety of your food. Use a hydrogen peroxide and water solution to wipe down your kitchen appliances like refrigerators, rice cookers, stoves, ovens, and dishwashers to remove stains and grime. You'll not only maintain their appearance but also keep them in good working condition longer.

Kitchen sponges, brushes, and towels are a favorite breeding ground of harmful bacteria which may spread from there to your plates, utensils, and other surfaces. You may soak them for 5-10 minutes in hydrogen peroxide to wash away food stains and keep them free of bacteria. Rinse well and allow them to air dry after soaking.

Pots and pans are often the hardest kitchen implements to clean. Remove stubborn food stains, oils, and residues on your pots and pans with a paste of baking soda and hydrogen peroxide. Scrub directly on your pots and pans, then let soak for a few minutes. Repeat this as necessary and then wash as usual.

Garden Uses

Many people have yet to discover that the garden is another part of home where hydrogen peroxide proves its versatility and comes in handy. It can be used in a wide variety of gardening styles, including planting directly in the ground, in pots or containers, and in raised beds. It is even used in hydroponics and greenhouses. It also works well for a wide range of plant varieties from flowers to fruit-bearing trees, vegetables, ornamentals, and other trees. Unless otherwise specified, you will need 3% hydrogen peroxide and water. With these simple-to-follow tips, you can use hydrogen peroxide to turn yourself into the ultimate green thumb.

- Soil Preparation – Spray your garden, potting soil, or garden patch with a few squirts of water and peroxide solution to ward of funguses, viruses, and bacteria that may affect the growth and health of your plants. This can also help keep away insects and other pests.

- Sprouting – Hydrogen peroxide can be used to effectively condition your sprouting seeds and prepare them for planting. Soak your sprouts in an 8% hydrogen peroxide water bath for three to four hours. This helps sprouts grow faster and healthier. It also helps protect your seed sprouts from mold and fungus.

- Rooting – Spray the roots of your plants with equal parts hydrogen peroxide and water before potting or ground planting. Doing so disinfects and protects them from disease, bacteria, insects, and fungus.

- Cuttings – Add hydrogen peroxide to your water bath for cuttings. Once they are planted, add hydrogen peroxide to the water you use to water them. This helps improve their health and aids in faster, stronger, and more productive growth.

- Natural Fertilizer – Use hydrogen peroxide as an all-natural fertilizer by adding a cup or two to the water you use to water your plants. This helps improve growth and overall plant health, and may also increase harvest or blooms of your fruiting and flowering plants.

- Natural Pesticide – Add equal parts of hydrogen peroxide to water and use in a spray bottle to apply to your plant's leaves and stems. This may help prevent insects and bugs from chomping on your greenery.

- Hydroponic Gardening – You may add hydrogen peroxide to your watering system as an additional source of protection and health aid for your hydroponic garden.

- Cleaning – As in your kitchen and other parts of your home, a hydrogen peroxide and water solution can serve as an all-around, all-purpose cleaner for your garden shed or greenhouse. It may also be used as a disinfectant and stain remover for your garden implements and tools. Use it like your usual cleaners.

Effects on Plant Health

Hydrogen peroxide is used by many farmers as an all-natural agricultural pesticide because of its ability to kill bacteria, pests and insects, parasites, mold, and fungi. Because it is an all-natural substance, it aids plant growth in an environmentally safe manner, eliminating risks of adverse chemical effects and run-off in the environment.

Ailing Plants

Whether the problem is fungus, blight, aphids, or pests, add a cup of hydrogen peroxide to water and use to spray or water your ailing plants daily. For severe cases, apply the peroxide full strength to affected leaves once or twice a week until your plant recovers.

Neglected Plants

Let's admit there may be times we tend to neglect our plants and forget to water them. Use half a cup of hydrogen peroxide with one gallon of water to water your plants and help them recover faster. But of course, make sure you don't over-water.

Hydrogen peroxide is a safe, economical, and all-natural product that works effectively for general all-purpose cleaning in all areas of our homes. Make sure, though, that you handle and use it with precaution as you would any other home cleaning aid.

Chapter 10:
Cool Experiments with Hydrogen Peroxide

Detection of fingerprints using hydrogen peroxide and vinegar

Materials

- 2 % or 3 % hydrogen peroxide
- White vinegar (5 % acetic acid)
- A brass item which has fingerprints
- Beaker
- Water wash
- Gloves

Procedure

1. Add 10 parts of 2 % or 3 % hydrogen peroxide to 7 parts of distilled white vinegar in a beaker.
2. Put a brass object which has hidden fingerprints into the beaker containing hydrogen peroxide.
3. Wait for around 5 to 10 minutes (until you see a green color around the brass object).
4. Decant the green-colored solution into another beaker.
5. Rinse the brass object with distilled water several times.

6. Dry the brass item using a tissue paper.

7. Now the brass object will have clearly visible fingerprints on it.

Caution: Always use gloves while handling hydrogen peroxide. If hydrogen peroxide falls on hands, it should be washed with plenty of running water.

The science behind the reaction is that the mixture of vinegar and acetic acid is acidic in nature and has a strong oxidizing capacity. Brass is an alloy of copper and some other metals. When copper is exposed to a strong oxidizing agent and an acid it reacts to form a copper salt, in this case copper acetate. However, the area that has fingerprints is coated with a layer of oil (as our fingers have oil on them), and so the copper beneath it cannot react with the acid or strong oxidizing agent and hence remains unchanged. This makes fingerprints clearly visible.

Reaction of hydrogen peroxide with blood

Materials

- 30 % hydrogen peroxide
- Blood (human or animal)
- Beaker
- Syringe
- Gloves

Procedure

1. Rinse the beaker with distilled water and let it dry.
2. Pour around 15 ml of 30 % hydrogen peroxide.
3. Pour a drop or two of blood.
4. Watch the magic.

Caution: Do not harm yourself, others or any animal to obtain blood. This experiment hould only be done under the supervision of adults. Always use gloves while handling hydrogen peroxide. If hydrogen peroxide falls on hands, it should be washed with plenty of running water.

The science behind this experiment is that blood has a large number of enzymes with varying functions. One such enzyme helps the blood to clot. This enzyme is activated when we are wounded. As we pour blood onto the hydrogen peroxide, the enzyme is activated and forms a clot (in the form of a thin layer on the surface of the hydrogen peroxide). Blood also has enzymes that catalyze the decomposition of water and oxygen. As soon as the clot is formed the oxygen produced does not have any way to go up, so it forms a blobby structure under the clotted layer. Isn't this awesome?

Hydrogen peroxide hybrid rocket

Materials

- Hydrogen peroxide, 30 % concentration
- Baker's yeast (*Saccharomyces cerevisiae*)
- Glass jar

- The metal lid of the glass jar
- Cylindrical pasta
- Cello tape
- Pair of scissors
- Matchbox
- Gloves

Procedure

1. Take the glass jar and its lid and clean them properly.
2. Make a hole of about the size of the pasta in the center of the lid and set it aside.
3. Fill the jar ¾ full with the hydrogen peroxide.
4. Add a teaspoon of yeast and mix it well in the hydrogen peroxide.
5. Close the lid immediately and seal it with cello tape. (Make sure that the seal is airtight).
6. Put the pasta in the hole in the lid of the jar.
7. Light the pasta with a matchstick and enjoy.

Caution: This experiment is a potential fire hazard and should only be performed outdoors under the supervision of adults. Always use gloves while handling hydrogen peroxide. If hydrogen peroxide falls on hands, it should be washed with plenty of running water.

The science behind the experiment is more biochemical than chemical. As discussed earlier, hydrogen peroxide has the ability to decompose. As it decomposes, it produces hydrogen gas and water. Since this process is slow, we add baker's yeast (*Saccharomyces cerevisiae*) to hasten it. Yeast is a living organism and has the ability to convert hydrogen peroxide into water and hydrogen gas faster than would normally occur; hence it is called a catalyst. In the packet, baker's yeast is in a dormant state; it becomes active when it comes into contact with water. *Saccharomyces cerevisiae* has an enzyme that catalyzes the reaction of hydrogen peroxide decomposition.

The pasta acts as a fuel and the oxygen gas produced enhances the combustion process. This is the basic concept of all hybrid rockets.

Making an oxygen balloon with hydrogen peroxide

Materials

- 5 mL hydrogen peroxide (30 % concentration)
- 10 mL bleach (the chosen bleach should have sodium hypochlorite)
- Test tube
- Balloon
- Funnel
- Gloves

Procedure

1. Take a test tube, clean it with distilled water, and let it dry.

2. Pour 10 mL of bleach in the test tube, using a funnel.

3. Put the funnel in the opening of the balloon and fill it with 5 mL of hydrogen peroxide.

4. Stretch the mouth of the balloon over the opening of the test tube.

5. Slowly pour the hydrogen peroxide from the balloon into the test tube.

6. As the reaction between the hydrogen peroxide and bleach proceeds, oxygen gas is formed, along with bubbles.

7. The released oxygen gas accumulates in the balloon.

Caution: When sealing the opening of the test tube with the balloon, be sure that the seal is airtight. Otherwise, the oxygen gas produced will escape and will not be collected in the balloon. The chosen bleach must contain sodium hypochlorite. Always use gloves while handling hydrogen peroxide. If hydrogen peroxide falls on hands, it should be washed with plenty of running water.

The science behind the reaction is that hydrogen peroxide can decompose in water and oxygen. As we add the bleach containing sodium hypochlorite, it acts as a catalyst and speeds up the decomposition reaction. As hydrogen peroxide decomposes, it forms oxygen and water. As oxygen is lighter than water, it is forced up into the balloon, and the balloon is filled with oxygen.

Explosive decomposition of hydrogen peroxide

Materials

- Hydrogen peroxide (30% concentration)
- Potassium iodide (KI)
- Measuring cylinder (100 mL)
- Conical flask
- Gloves
- Filter paper
- Protective eye gear

Procedure

1. Take a 100 mL measuring cylinder and clean it.
2. Put approximately 50 mL of the hydrogen peroxide in the measuring cylinder.
3. Pour the peroxide into a conical flask.
4. Take a clean filter paper and put approximately 5 grams of potassium iodide (KI) in it. Fold the filter paper such that the potassium iodide is not exposed to the atmosphere.

5. Drop the packet of potassium iodide into the conical flask containing the hydrogen peroxide.

6. Quickly move back from the conical flask and enjoy the show.

Caution: The conical flask must be made of thick glass. Do not forget to wear gloves and protective eye gear. Potassium iodide must be packed with care.

The science behind the reaction is that hydrogen peroxide can decompose to water and oxygen gas. The added potassium iodide acts as a catalyst and speeds up the reaction. The reason why potassium iodide has to be packed in filter paper is because the catalytic reaction is so vigorous that it might occur immediately and spill on the face of the person performing the experiment. Another function of potassium iodide is that it imparts a cool color to the hydrogen peroxide bubbles. If hydrogen peroxide falls on hands, it should be washed with plenty of running water.

Elephant toothpaste

Materials

- Measuring cylinder
- Hydrogen peroxide, 30 % concentration
- Potassium iodide (KI) or manganese oxide (MnO_2)
- Gloves
- Liquid detergent
- Plastic bottle

- Protective eye gear

Procedure

1. Take a measuring cylinder and clean it with water.

2. Measure 200 mL of hydrogen peroxide.

3. Pour the peroxide into a plastic bottle.

4. Add up to 10 mL of liquid detergent to it.

5. Shake the bottle well to mix the detergent and the hydrogen peroxide.

6. Put up to 15 gm of potassium iodide (KI) or manganese oxide (MnO_2) in a test tube.

7. Add water to the test tube containing potassium iodide (KI) or manganese oxide (MnO_2) and make a solution.

8. Slowly add the solution to the bottle containing the hydrogen peroxide and detergent mixture.

9. Step back and enjoy.

Note: Food coloring can also be added to the mixture of hydrogen peroxide and detergent to give the elephant toothpaste a color.

Caution: The potassium iodide or manganese dioxide should be carefully packed in a filter paper to avoid an overly quick reaction. The detergent used should not hinder the catalysis of the hydrogen peroxide. Wear gloves and protective eye gear to be safe from the chemicals used. If hydrogen peroxide falls on hands, it should be washed with plenty of running water.

The science behind the reaction is that KI and MnO$_2$ are very good catalysts for converting hydrogen peroxide into water and oxygen. The foamy texture of the elephant toothpaste is due to the detergent used in the reaction. If the hydrogen peroxide is concentrated, the toothpaste shoots out from the bottle like a rocket.

The color-changing rose

Materials

- Red rose with a short stem
- Sulfur powder
- Hydrogen peroxide, 30 % concentration
- Matchbox
- Aluminum foil
- Beakers (two)
- Cello tape

Procedure

1. Take the beakers and clean them.
2. Take the rose and stick it on the side of one of the beakers with the cello tape, such that the rose faces the bottom of the beaker. (Make sure that the rose does not touch the bottom of the beaker.)
3. Put the aluminum foil on the ground and put some sulfur on it.

4. Light the sulfur with a match. Let the sulfur burn until you can smell it.

5. Take the beaker with the rose and cover the burning sulfur with it. Make sure that the rose petals are completely exposed to the sulfur dioxide fumes.

6. Leave it in the same position for about 15 minutes.

7. Remove the rose from the beaker and put it in the second beaker.

8. Pour hydrogen peroxide into it until the rose is completely submerged.

9. Watch the rose carefully and note your observations.

Caution: Wear gloves and protective eye gear while handling hydrogen peroxide. Do not inhale sulfur dioxide fumes.

I hope you have enjoyed the reasoning behind the previous experiments – now it's your turn to understand the science by yourself.

Hint: Hydrogen peroxide does not decompose in this reaction.

Chapter 11:
Precautions and Safe Practices

In order for you to get the most out of hydrogen peroxide, you need to know a few crucial guiding principles to ensure that you can safely avoid minor or even fatal injury. First, you need to understand the different grades of hydrogen peroxide and their conventional uses. When buying hydrogen peroxide, you need to confirm that it is a suitable grade for the specific use you're planning.

Grades of Hydrogen Peroxide

Pharmaceutical grade hydrogen peroxide – 3.5% concentration: this is the type that is available at your local drugstore or supermarket. This grade of hydrogen peroxide is not recommended for internal use since it contains a selection of stabilizers that should not be ingested, including carbolic acid, acetanilide, tetrasodium pyrophosphate, and sodium stannate.

- Beautician Grade Hydrogen peroxide – 6% concentration: this type is often used in beauty and cosmetic applications, and it is definitely not recommended for internal use.

- Laboratory Grade Hydrogen Peroxide – 30% concentration: this concentration of hydrogen peroxide is employed in the laboratory for a variety of scientific research and experiments. This grade also includes stabilizers and internal use is prohibited.

- Electronic Grade Hydrogen Peroxide – Between 30% and 32% concentration: this grade of hydrogen peroxide is applied in the cleaning of electronic parts. It is never to be used internally.

- Technical Grade Hydrogen Peroxide – 35% concentration: this hydrogen peroxide grade contains added phosphorous that helps in the neutralization of any chlorine present in the water with which it is diluted.

- Food Grade Hydrogen Peroxide – 35% concentration: this is the only grade of hydrogen peroxide that is recommended and approved for internal use. It is used in production of food products that contain eggs, cheese, and whey. This grade of hydrogen peroxide is also sprayed on the lining foil of aseptic packages that contain milk products and fruit juices.

- Fuel Grade Hydrogen Peroxide – 90% concentration: this astounding concentration of hydrogen peroxide is used as a source of oxygen in rocket fuel.

Dilution of Hydrogen Peroxide

Since hydrogen peroxide is highly reactive with almost any element that comes in contact with it, it is crucial that you dilute it only with distilled water. Distilled water is extremely purified water that is free of any contaminants or impurities. Impurities can lead to a very rapid reaction when water gets into contact with hydrogen peroxide. For example, tap water typically contains several mineral salts that are accompanied by a combination of complex chemicals. These chemicals can react with hydrogen peroxide in very destructive ways that can lead to injury. In addition, bottled water often contains mineral salts that are added to increase its nutritional value, and can also react vigorously upon contact with hydrogen peroxide. To prevent all these unexpected and dangerous reactions, use only pure water to dilute hydrogen peroxide.

To ensure purity, buy a water purifier and a TDS (Total Dissolved Solids) meter kit. A TDS meter kit is a very convenient piece of equipment that will measure the total electrical conductivity of your water and give you a precise indication of the amount of contamination. It is actually rather cheap and relatively easy to use.

When diluting concentrated hydrogen peroxide, keep the following in mind:

- Use a very clean, sterile Pyrex® or glass container or graduated cylinder.

- Wear full protective gear, basically gloves and safety goggles, in case of any spills.

- Avoid any skin contact with concentrated hydrogen peroxide; in case of contact, flush thoroughly with a generous amount of water.

Dilution from 35% hydrogen peroxide

Dilution to a concentration of 3% hydrogen peroxide

- 11 parts of distilled water
- 1 part of 35% hydrogen peroxide solution

Dilution to a 6% concentration of hydrogen peroxide

- 11 parts of distilled water
- 2 parts of 35% hydrogen peroxide solution

Storage and Decomposition of Hydrogen Peroxide

The rate at which hydrogen peroxide decomposes into its basic byproducts, oxygen and water, is not constant as it is dependent upon a variety of factors. Exposure to heat and/or light dramatically accelerates the process of decomposition. Hydrogen peroxide products sold for domestic uses tend to be rather unstable. That is, they easily decompose to the more stable oxygen and water molecules.

On the other hand, the industrial and technical grade hydrogen peroxide products often have stabilizing additives that tend to slow down this breakdown. However, be careful not to contaminate them, as this can lead to more rapid decomposition. This reaction will weaken the solution through the breakdown of hydrogen peroxide and the formation of byproducts.

Storage

- Store your hydrogen peroxide in a cool, dry place that is adequately ventilated to prevent accumulation of heat. Keep it in the original manufacturer's container, and make sure that young children cannot access it.
- Although heat speeds up the decomposition process, this does not mean that hydrogen peroxide must be stored in a refrigerator, and it should not be frozen.

Besides, storing it in a refrigerator puts it close to any infants or toddlers in your household, which is a potentially hazardous situation.

- Storing hydrogen peroxide in glass containers is not generally recommended, since they may contain trace amounts of alkaline ions of metals. However, glass containers with coated interiors may be used, as the coating prevents any reaction between the hydrogen peroxide and the walls of the container.

- The storage container should always be kept in an upright position to avoid spills.

- Hydrogen peroxide begins to decompose when it is exposed to light, so keep it in containers that are either dark or tinted.

- Make sure the container you use has an airtight seal to prevent any atmospheric contamination.

Basic Safety Precautions When Using Hydrogen Peroxide

- Ensure that you wash your hands thoroughly after using it, however briefly.

- Rinse fresh fruits and vegetables thoroughly after disinfecting them with hydrogen peroxide.

- Always follow any instructions on the container.

First Aid

Hydrogen peroxide can produce quite a number of potentially harmful or fatal effects, so you need to know how to deal with the dangers of exposure. The first aid to be employed in specific situations depends on the grade of hydrogen peroxide involved. Some situations will require immediate medical attention; in others home remedies will suffice.

- Inhalation – If someone inhales hydrogen peroxide, immediately move him or her to a place with plenty of fresh air, preferably an open space. A well-ventilated interior area would also be appropriate. If the person is not breathing, give any form of artificial respiration, if possible the mouth-to-mouth technique. If he or she is breathing with difficulty, provide an adequate supply of oxygen and contact a medical practitioner or paramedic immediately.

- Contact with the Eyes – If you get hydrogen peroxide in your eyes, immediately flush them with lots of clean water for a minimum of fifteen minutes, periodically raising both the upper and lower lids. If you were wearing contact lenses, remove them immediately. Figure out whether your vision has been affected, which would indicate more extensive damage that requires the attention of an ophthalmologist.

- Contact with the skin – If any amount of concentrated hydrogen peroxide spills on your skin, flush the point of contact immediately with a lot of clean water for a minimum of fifteen minutes. Also remove all contaminated clothing (and even shoes) to prevent further irritation. If there are any obvious burns, seek medical help from a physician.

- Ingestion or swallowing – if you accidentally swallow or ingest hydrogen peroxide, you should NEVER try to induce emesis (vomiting). Instead, drink about four to eight ounces of fresh milk or water. If you are dealing with an unconscious victim of hydrogen peroxide ingestion, do not give him or her anything to drink. Seek medical assistance immediately.

Firefighting Measures Related to Hydrogen Peroxide

Hydrogen peroxide is a Class 2 oxidizer which, while not flammable itself, undergoes thermal decomposition that produces heat and oxygen. This process greatly increases the potential for combustion or explosion of flammable vapors with which it comes in contact. Hydrogen peroxide can also decompose certain other compounds, leading to the production of hazardous fumes.

Instructions for fighting a fire involving hydrogen peroxide:

1. Firefighters should wear full protective equipment, including a self-contained breathing apparatus.

2. Use only water to extinguish the fire, as any other fire extinguishing agent may end up reacting with the hydrogen peroxide and making the situation worse.

3. Also use water to cool containers that have been exposed to the fire.

4. The area affected by the fire should be generously flooded with water.

Hydrogen peroxide's many advantages make it very important to our daily lives. If you know the proper precautions for using it, you can safely enjoy its uncountable merits – from internal health to external beautification and nourishing benefits. Are all at your disposal as long as you know how to deal with it carefully and appropriately. If you don't, you might find yourself in very some destructive situations!

Conclusion

Thank you for downloading this book!

It has truly been a delight to introduce you to the wonders of hydrogen peroxide. I have striven to make this book as relevant and insightful as possible. I hope the simple, step-by-step guidelines you've learned here have opened a whole new world for you and encouraged you to discover and experience for yourself how this wonder substance works.

I have done my best to make this book the most comprehensive and authoritative – yet simple – guide to practical home uses for hydrogen peroxide. I focused on the benefits of using hydrogen peroxide for health and wellness because I believe good health should be the foundation of how we live our lives.

I hope to encourage many more people to explore and enjoy the many uses and benefits of hydrogen peroxide and how it can be used to improve and protect your overall health and well-being. Take advantage of this natural, environmentally safe, economical, and versatile wonder to help you achieve and maintain a better quality of life for you and your loved ones.

With a can-do attitude, I invite you to go ahead and discover and explore the many ways hydrogen peroxide can work for you! If you come up with your own ingenuous way to use hydrogen peroxide at home, I hope you'll share it with me for inclusion in an expanded sequel to this work.

I would love to hear feedback from you on how using this book has helped you in your everyday life.

Key Takeaways

- Hydrogen peroxide is a naturally occurring substance composed of hydrogen and water.

- Hydrogen peroxide is a powerful disinfectant that kills harmful organisms through oxidation.

- Hydrogen peroxide is economical and environmentally safe.

- Hydrogen peroxide can be safely used at home for various beauty applications, health treatments, and all-around home applications.

- Learn how to safely use hydrogen peroxide to benefit your health and for various applications at home.

- Using hydrogen peroxide at home mostly requires 3% H_2O_2 and water.

- Hydrogen peroxide, when used properly and appropriately, helps promote overall health and wellness and a better quality of life.

How to Put This Information into Action

This book explains the nature of hydrogen peroxide: what it is made of, how it works, why it is beneficial, and how we can harness its properties to benefit our health and overall wellness as well as improve our way of life. It is important to begin with this explanation because understanding the nature of any substance is important to truly appreciating its properties. Once we understand something better, we are able to let go of our preconceived notions and prejudices. Removing these barriers encourages us and allows us to try out new things. A true understanding of what hydrogen peroxide is can help encourage us to start using it or use it more often, and even inspire innovation and improvisation in its use. Also, knowing the nature of hydrogen peroxide enables us to better understand how to use it safely, without risk to anyone, and without adversely affecting the environment.

- Chapter 3 – From the first discovery of this compound, a lot has been done to ensure that it is absolutely safe for use. All the insight gained from both its physical and chemical properties should make you really appreciate the revolutionary work of the eminent scientists responsible for its discovery, isolation, and mass production. Without them, it is likely that our lives would have been rather more difficult. Even today, experiments are still being performed on both domestic and industrial uses of this amazing compound. All the facts and figures from this in-depth research will make it even easier to incorporate hydrogen peroxide into your regular undertakings. They give you the information on how to use it and how not to use it, as well as what to do in case there is an accident.

- Chapter 7 – With the uncountable scientifically backed merits of hydrogen peroxide, it is quite clear that its regular use will thoroughly boost your overall nourishment and help in reinforcing of the body's immunity. You should follow the guidelines strictly, especially in intravenous administration and bath therapy, as excessive concentrations are prone to have negative effects. If you have a prescription from a doctor, stick to it! Furthermore, plants health can also be maintained by using this exceptional compound to enhance sustenance and cure oxygen deficiency disorders. Precision in concentrations and measurements is equally significant in plant care.

- Chapter 8 – This chapter presents easy-to-follow steps for using materials found in most homes to harness hydrogen peroxide for beauty applications. It is divided into sections on specific body areas, making it easier to refer to a particular application when you need it. The chapter also includes useful tips and tricks to help enhance the beauty effects of hydrogen peroxide. The section on hair care in particular is a comprehensive, yet easy-to-follow how-to on achieving the perfect bleached look. It is intended to enable you to economically and easily apply one of the most popular hair coloring compounds with confidence and peace of mind.

- Chapter 9 – Achieving overall wellness and maintaining good health and a healthy lifestyle must always begin at home. No health and beauty regimen is ever effective if one's immediate surroundings are not conducive to healthy habits and practices. The use of hydrogen peroxide in our homes may contribute greatly to creating a space for rest and relaxation. Maintaining healthy living conditions is an integral part of living a healthy lifestyle. The chapter presents easy-to-follow steps and uses materials we all have at home. The section on gardening presents some of the simplest gardening applications for hydrogen peroxide; while many sources list various methods for using hydrogen peroxide in the garden, I have included here only the easiest methods with the least need for specialized tools and equipment.

- Chapter 11 – When using hydrogen peroxide, it is absolutely better to be safe than sorry, all the way from buying it, through using it, to storing it. When buying it at a supermarket or pharmacy, be sure to confirm its concentration (percentage of hydrogen peroxide) is appropriate for what you want to use it for. It is also crucial to follow the easy steps for safe handling and dilution (if necessary). Proper storage will keep it from abrupt decomposition and prevent unnecessary accidents. If there is an accident, use the first aid guidelines given to provide immediate treatment, and then consult a medical practitioner.

Hydrogen peroxide can work for you to improve most aspects of your home life. An optimistic spirit coupled with a little common sense can go a long way in helping you take advantage of this liquid elixir. Most of the materials you need can be found right in your own home, so there's no need to go out of your way to buy new things for your hydrogen peroxide applications. Use the knowledge you gained from this book as a foundation for coming up with more creative ways to use hydrogen peroxide. You may use this book as your handy go-to manual for your everyday hydrogen peroxide applications.

Feel free to make your own notes and record the ratios for your solutions and variations in your applications as you go along. This book is designed to give you the freedom to customize the ways you use hydrogen peroxide to truly address your unique needs and preferences.

Don't forget to take the necessary safety precautions when doing your applications! Handling hydrogen peroxide safely is not rocket science and doesn't require a biohazard suit. A little common sense and a healthy respect for safety procedures can go a long way toward allowing you to enjoy the benefits of this wonder substance safely. So embrace the possibilities, and you are well on your way to reaping the benefits and rewards of using hydrogen peroxide.

Resources for Further Reading and Viewing

http://kimiainternational.com/hydrogen-peroxide/

http://www.wikihow.com/Bleach-Your-Hair-With-Hydrogen-Peroxide

http://www.realfarmacy.com/20-benefits-and-uses-for-hydrogen-peroxide/

http://www.sore-throat-remedies.com/hydrogen-peroxide-for-a-sore-throat/

http://www.ehow.com/facts_6370209_hydrogen-peroxide-skin-care.html

http://www.livestrong.com/article/511371-how-to-use-hydrogen-peroxide-on-acne-skin/

https://www.facebook.com/101homeusesofhydrogenperoxide

http://www.ehow.com/facts_5907933_hydrogen-peroxide-nail-fungus.html

http://www.care2.com/greenliving/15-surprising-uses-for-hydrogen-peroxide.html

http://wakeup-world.com/2012/07/09/27-amazing-benefits-and-uses-for-hydrogen-peroxide/

http://www.purehealthsystems.com/hydrogen-peroxide-2.html

http://www.atsdr.cdc.gov/MMG/MMG.asp?id=304&tid=55

http://www.youtube.com/watch?v=vXWXhp6aFuw

http://educate-yourself.org/cancer/benefitsofhydrogenperozide17jul03.shtml

http://www.truthorfiction.com/rumors/h/hydrogen-peroxide.htm#.U8o1dvmSxmw

Preview of Natural Remedies that Work: How to Heal and Protect Yourself without the Use of Prescription

Chapter 2. Natural Remedies for Common Health Problems

The following are common health problems that affect us from time to time, and the natural remedies that we recommend.

Toothache

One of the most unpleasant experiences we can ever imagine is to suffer from a toothache. Toothaches affect us once in a while, even if we try to keep a good dental hygiene. The severity of the toothache may differ depending on the cause and extent of the problem. Normally a toothache warrants a visit to the dentist, but before you go there, you could use some remedy to alleviate the excruciating pain.

Clove oil

Clove oil is particularly effective in reducing the pain. It has antiseptic and germicidal properties that helps relieve toothaches. Clove oil contains eugenol, which has been used in dentistry for many years. To use, put a few drops of clove oil in a cotton ball and place it on the affected tooth.

Onion and Garlic

Onions and garlic too have been used by ancient cultures in dealing with toothaches. Crush a few cloves of garlic and a small onion bulb in a bowl and place on the bad tooth. They contain a substance known as allicin, which works as an anesthetic.

Oats

Oats too are very effective in soothing painful gums and teeth. They serve to drain out pus if present. Bite some oats with the side of the jaw having the painful teeth and hold down the crushed oats for around 10 minutes. You can then rinse your mouth with salty water. Salty water in itself can also be used for minor tooth and gum pains.

Bad Breath

Bad breath is a very common problem. In fact, most people have suffered from this at one point in their lives. Bad breath in most cases is not a health issue warranting a visit to the doctor. In a few cases though, where it persists, it can be a sign of deeper health problems.

Generally, bad breath is caused by teeth infections, gum sores, dehydration, sinus problems, smoking, high protein foods, stress, and some prescription medication among many other issues. Bad breath is very embarrassing and can cause one to have low self-esteem. Take heart, as there are natural ways to deal with bad breath.

Tea Tree Oil

Tea tree oil is great in fighting bad breath. It has antibacterial, antimicrobial and antiseptic properties, which aid in the cleaning of the oral cavity and removal of bad breath. Add a few drops of this oil to your toothbrush every time you brush your teeth. Tea tree oil can also be used as a mouthwash by adding three drops of the oil to warm water then gargling. Additionally, fresh fruit juices are a good way to fight bad breath.

Foot Odor

This is another major issue affecting many people especially men. There is often a misconception that smelly feet are a result of poor hygiene habits. This is not the case. Some people actually have a medical condition known as bromhidrosis, which is responsible for the bad odor. As with bad breath, smelly feet can cause someone to suffer from low self-esteem.

Foot odor starts when feet that are covered by socks and shoes develop a moist environment. This is where bacteria thrive. It might sound horrible, but it's possible to fight these bacteria using natural remedies. Finding a quality pair of socks that keep your feet dry is the first step. You can even find shoes that let the feet breath.

The following are the natural remedies that can cure foot odor:

Kosher Salt

Most salts have a drying effect on the skin, like the one we experience after a swim in the ocean. However, kosher salt is very good in absorbing moisture and odor. Add a good amount of it in some basin water and wash your feet. Do not mix with other detergents; it would be better if you did so after taking a bath. Do not rinse your feet after washing; rather, dry them thoroughly with a towel. This will serve to keep your feet dry for longer.

Baking Soda

This is a good deodorizing agent for your shoes. It has antimicrobial and anti-itch properties that protect the feet from infections. Sprinkle some baking soda into your shoes after removing them. Cornstarch too has the same effect.

Vinegar

This is used in the household as a superior cleaning agent and an odor fighting and deodorizing agent. When it comes to the feet, it actually helps too. Add ½ cup of vinegar to a bowl of water and soak your feet for 20 minutes. Do this once a week.

Ginger

Ginger has also been used in some regions to heal smelly feet, as it is a great disinfecting agent. Mash up some gingers, put the pulp into a handkerchief, and then soak it in warm water. Now rub the ginger liquid onto your feet every evening.

Fevers

Fevers are not a bad thing at all. It might sound contradictory because they make us feel terrible. Actually, fever is a sign that the body is fighting disease-causing organisms. The body raises its core temperature to kill organisms which won't survive the heat. However, fevers can get extremely bad that they warrant medical attention. One thing to note with fevers is that you shouldn't try covering yourself in bed, because you'll end up feeling much uncomfortable. Always take in a lot of water while having a fever to replace the water lost through sweating.

The following fruits and herbs are some of the natural remedies proven to cure fever:

Pineapples

Pineapples have been used successfully over the years to fight fevers. It is rich in Vitamin C and B6, folate and riboflavin. These are effective in flushing toxins out of your body and help you feel better. These fruits also have lots of water that will keep you hydrated all along.

Raisins

Raisins are known to fight fevers. It is rich in Phenolic Phytonutrients that is known for their germicidal, antibiotic and antioxidant properties. Chop around three quarters of a cup of raisins and add 7 cups of water. Boil them and let simmer. Take this water several times in a day to fight your fever.

Blackberry Vinegar

Blackberry vinegar is an effective remedy in treating fevers. Blackberries are rich in vitamins and minerals, and are a very potent antioxidant which will make you feel refreshed and rejuvenated. In fact, many cultures used it in the olden times. However, it requires some time to prepare. So its best prepared early when fever symptoms are noted. You need to have cider vinegar and blackberries. Pour some cider vinegar over the berries and cover the container for 2-3 days, then strain the liquid from these berries. Add some good amount of sugar to this mix. Then bring to a boil and finally simmer for 5 minutes. Store this mixture in a cool place. Take 1 teaspoonful and add in a cup of water.

Basil

Basil is another natural remedy for fevers. It relieves pain, and has antibacterial properties as well. Mix a teaspoonful of crushed basil with ¼ teaspoon of pepper. Put in a hot cup of water and you can add some honey. Drink it one of two times in a day.

Fruits

When experiencing a fever, most fruits are good at this time due to their vitamins and minerals, and their overall hydrating effect. Take a lot of fruits. Apples, oranges, lemons, and natural fruit juices will all work to reduce the effects of the fever.

Back Pain

Back pain is another common problem. Once in a while we all get to strain our backs. This is caused by several reasons such as carrying heavy loads, strenuous physical activity, old age, and sitting for an extended amount of time, among others. The bad thing with back pain is that your doctor cannot do much, other than prescribe painkillers for you and some rest. So why not try out some natural home remedies that will alleviate this pain?

It's important to take note that the back is extremely important in keeping us fit and moving. So adopt an upright sitting position. Walk with your back straight and if possible strengthen it with a few exercises. Swimming is the best exercise for your back.

If you have injured your back, put some ice on the painful area. This is mostly to avoid inflammation and decrease the pain. The best way to do this would be to put some ice in a paper bag, then put a towel on your back before placing the ice. Keep replacing the ice bag after every 15 minutes. Getting some rest is an old way of dealing with back pain especially one that was caused by strenuous physical activity. A massage will also come in handy. Chamomile tea is very effective in providing a calming effect which soothes tense muscles.

Burns

Burns are classified by degree. There are first, second and third degree burns. Most burns that we get at home are first degree burns. These are the type that affects just the outer layer of the skin. They are painful and cause redness. Burns affecting just a small area of the skin will be effectively treated at home. However, if a large part of the skin is covered by the burn at a vital area of the body such as the face is affected, then you might want to seek immediate medical attention.

Honey

For natural home remedies, honey is very effective in managing burns and wounds. Honey will draw out water from the blistered skin thus cleaning the wound. Apply honey directly to the wound. If the burn is in the mouth, then a salty water gargle will be helpful.

Milk

Milk is also effective in soothing a burn. After you suffer a burn and experience the hotness and pains, take in some cold milk, or dab it on the affected area with a cloth and wrap it. If it's a finger or the hand, dip it in milk as you would do with water; it's much more effective.

With burns, the best way is to avoid them as much as possible. If you have kids, discourage them from going to the kitchen when meals are being prepared.

Hangovers

Everybody who drinks alcohol has experienced a hangover. The hangovers range from the mild ones like a dizziness, to the very severe ones like extreme body pains. People normally take over the counter drugs to deal with these hangovers, but this is not necessary. Hangovers are caused by dehydration and alcohol toxins. Alcohol is a strong dehydrating agent, and after a night out partying, your body is left with less than the adequate amount of body water. This is what causes the dizziness, headaches and muscle aches.

Refreshing Fluids

The best remedy for a hangover is water. Take several glasses of water to hydrate the body.

Other natural products that fight hangovers are coconut water, honey and lemon drink, ginger ale, and boiled eggs. Avoid strongly flavored fluids as they may escalate the problem.

Fruits

Fruits are very effective too. Eat mostly bananas, as they replace potassium which was lost when drinking.

Asparagus

Asparagus is a remedy for hangovers too. It acts by reducing the amount of free radicals caused by the breakdown of alcohol, thus helping the liver in cleaning up the mess caused by alcohol. Asparagus can be consumed in many different ways and it would be much helpful if you did it before taking alcohol. Though even after drinking, it will still work. An extract of asparagus, asparagus supplest, or asparagus teas will all be effective.

There are a few things that you shouldn't do when having a hangover, though. Never drink coffee the morning after, as it will just dehydrate you further. Never take painkillers to heal a hangover, as they don't work and will just add more work to the already overworked liver. Do not drink more alcohol to deal with a hangover. The sickening effect may temporarily disappear but will come back stronger, and this is a sure way to start alcohol addiction.

Nausea

Nausea is a pretty common problem that afflicts us once in a while. It can be caused by a certain food we have eaten, or can be a sign of a deeper lying problem in our bodies. In most cases however, it's not a big deal and can be dealt with by natural products at home. These remedies are meant to ease on the sickening feeling. Is symptoms persist and become severe, seek medical assistance for a full diagnosis.

Refreshing Fluids

Take water or other clear fluids like coconut water to hydrate the body. Avoid strongly flavored fluids such as overly-sweet fruit juices as they may escalate the problem.

Milk

Milk is a good nausea-fighting agent. Drink a glass of warm milk and take a rest. If unable to eat cooked foods, take a toast and crumble it in milk and eat. This is a vintage milk toast that has been used for nauseating patients.

Aniseed

Aniseed helps cure nausea. Brew some aniseed by placing ¼ teaspoon in half a cup of water. Steep for around 5 minutes and strain. You can also sprinkle aniseed onto cooked vegetables.

Mint Tea

Mild nausea can be dealt with by drinking mint tea. It cures the kind of nausea that comes by eating some types of food. Drink mint tea the normal way you drink your tea.

Stress

We all experience stress, only some people may have more than others. In fact, stress is not a bad thing; it's just the body's way of subconsciously protecting itself by increasing its response to potentially harmful situations. We all go though stressful periods in our life: be they work, family, or heath.

However, when stress has become chronic, it becomes a problem which can lead to depression. The good thing is that minor stresses in life are effectively dealt with by natural remedies which we are going to discuss here. These are meant to relax the mind.

Baking Soda and Ginger

A bath in baking soda and ginger has a soothing effect on the body which reduces stress. So next time you get home from work feeling all stressed up, add 1/3 cup of baking soda in your bath water and take a long bath to relive all the built up stress.

Lettuce

Also known as the stress-reducing vegetable, it has a sedative effect due to the presence of lacturcarium. So anytime you feel stressed, include lettuce in your meal.

Celery

Celery has the same effect as lettuce due to the presence of phthalides which are natural sedatives.

Oatmeal

Oatmeal has been used to fight off stress. Oats are highly nutritious and have been known to be very effective in fighting cholesterol. Consume a bowl in any way you fancy them.

Memory Loss Problems

Memory loss is normal and affects a big part of our population. Forgetting where you placed something, the names of people, or a certain event is something we all have experienced. When it happens repeatedly, then it becomes a problem. This could be at times embarrassing. If the memory loss is not caused by an underlying medical condition like Alzheimer, then the following natural remedies will improve your memory to a great extent.

Wheat Germ

Wheat germ is a very good source of vitamin E which greatly aids in boosting memory.

Pistachio Nuts

This kind of nut is full of thiamine, which is useful in assisting memory especially for older people.

Memory Enhancing Foods

Other foods known to improve memory are carrots, eggs, okra and blueberries.

[Click here to download the rest of this book.](#)

More Books You Might Like

Household DIY: Save Time and Money with Do It Yourself Hints and Tips on Furniture, Clothes, Pests, Stains, Residues, Odors and More!

DIY Household Hacks: Save Time and Money with Do It Yourself Tips and Tricks for Cleaning Your House

Essential Oils: Essential Oils & Aromatherapy for Beginners: Proven Secrets to Weight Loss, Skin Care, Hair Care & Stress Relief Using Essential Oil Recipes

Apple Cider Vinegar for Beginners: An Apple Cider Vinegar Handbook with Proven Secrets to Natural Weight Loss, Optimum Health and Beautiful Skin

Body Butter Recipes: Proven Formula Secrets to Making All Natural Body Butters that Will Hydrate and Rejuvenate Your Skin

If the links do not work, for whatever reason, you can simply search for these titles on the Amazon website to find them.

Your Free Bonus

As a way of thanking you for your purchase, I'm offering you an opportunity to sign up and be a part of an exclusive book list where members get advanced notice on high-quality books.

To be part of this exclusive club, click on the link below:

https://docs.google.com/forms/d/1ttDqtdRjOeAEtA-BKnq5Hw668vjQS0VWcXCGQ8z9frA/viewform

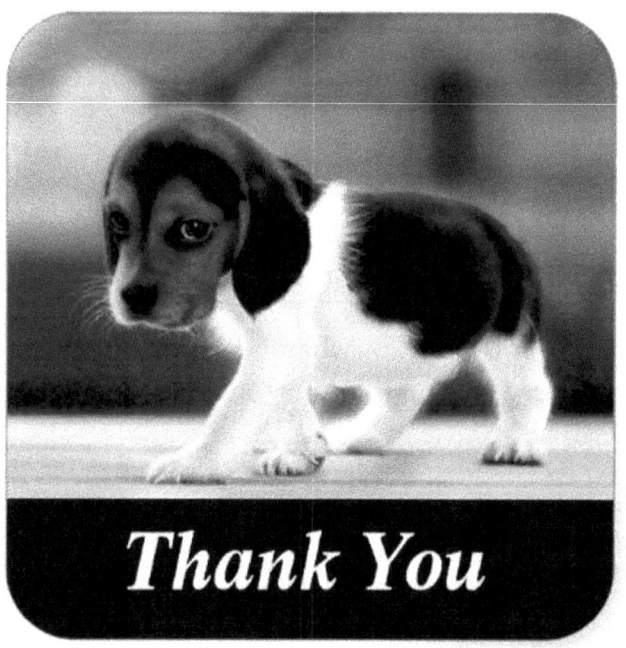

www.ingramcontent.com/pod-product-compliance
Lightning Source LLC
LaVergne TN
LVHW020350260326
834688LV00045B/1632